D0951937

ANNE HOOPER'S

POCKET

KAMA
SUTRA

*A new guide to the ancient
arts of love*

A DK PUBLISHING BOOK

Created and produced by
CARROLL & BROWN LIMITED
5 Lonsdale Road
London NW6 6RA

Project Editor Ian Wood
Designer Karen Sawyer
Production Wendy Rogers

First American Edition, 1996
20

Published in the United States by
DK Publishing, Inc., 375 Hudson St.
New York, New York 10014

A catalog record is available from the Library of Congress.

ISBN 0-7894-0437-0

Reproduced by Colourscan, Singapore
Printed and bound in Italy by LEGO

see our complete product line at **www.dk.com**

CONTENTS

INTRODUCTION

The Kama Sutra *was written for the nobility of India by a nobleman, Vatsyayana, at some time between* A.D. 100 *and* A.D. 400. *In those days, the typical*

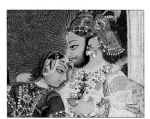

Indian nobleman led a life of leisured luxury and had ample free time to devote, if he so wished, to learning and perfecting the social, sexual, and artistic skills described in books such as the Kama Sutra.

The ideal citizen was supposed to dedicate his life to the achievement of three goals: *dharma* (the acquisition of religious merit), *artha* (acquisition of wealth), and *kama* (acquisition of love or sensual pleasure). The *Kama Sutra* was intended to help with the third of these goals—in discussing them, Vatsyayana says that "Kama is to be learned from the *Kama Sutra* and from the practice of citizens."

These three goals have their modern counterparts. Many of us aren't so enthusiastic about religious merit, but we do seek personal growth and fulfillment;

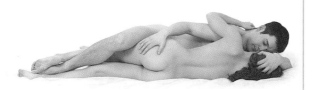

most of us do not aspire to great wealth, but do hope for enough money to live comfortably; and most of us want a loving sexual relationship.

The *Kama Sutra* was aimed at men (women were very much subordinate to them then), but that isn't to say that it ignores the needs of women—it doesn't. For example, it gives explicit instructions on female stimulation, including the advice that the "work of a man" includes kissing and stroking, and, if a woman is left unsatisfied by the act of intercourse, Vatsyayana recommends that "the man should rub the yoni [vulva] of the woman with his hand." He also advocates specific sexual positions to suit the physical match of

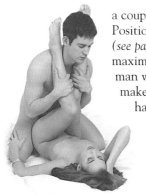

a couple. For instance, the Position of the Wife of Indra (*see page 64*) permits the maximum penetration when a man with a small lingam [penis] makes love to a woman who has a deep vagina. The Twining Position, on the other hand (*see page 68*), allows easy penetration when a man has a large penis and his partner a small vagina.

I have based this illustrated version of the *Kama Sutra* on the classic translation by Sir Richard Burton and F. F. Arbuthnot (first published in 1883). This version includes, alongside those parts of the original book that are still relevant, some other chunks of Vatsyayana's 2,000-year-old text because what these passages describe is in fascinating contrast to our sexual lives today.

In general, this book concentrates on foreplay and lovemaking and, of course, on the sexual positions for which the *Kama Sutra* has become famous. I have also, where I thought it necessary or helpful, supplemented the original information with suggestions and comments of my own.

For example, I have included information on safer sex, which, unfortunately, is all too necessary today. And because the use of a condom is often essential, whether for contraception or for safer sex, I have suggested ways to make it an erotic part of lovemaking rather than a chore. Also included is a section on sensual massage (*see pages 28–33*), which was not mentioned in the original but is a wonderful way to begin lovemaking.

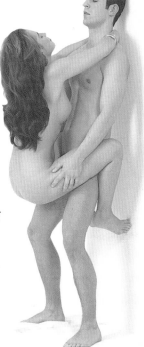

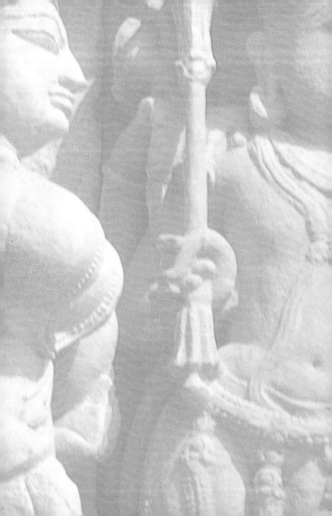

SETTING THE SCENE

"In all these things connected with love, everybody should act according to his own inclination."

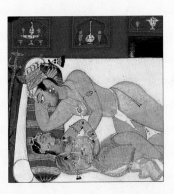

PREPARING THE BODY

In its description of the "life of a citizen," the Kama Sutra sets out a program of personal hygiene that is to be followed "without fail." This program includes cleaning the teeth, eating betel leaves and other things that sweeten the breath, bathing daily, and applying oils and perfumes to the body. The book's author, Vatsyayana, clearly understood the need for cleanliness, and most lovers today—just like those in ancient India—regard it as essential.

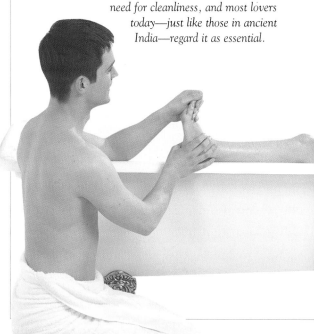

PERFUMING THE BREATH

Passion is easily dampened by body odor, and body odor combined with bad breath can destroy it completely; fortunately, deodorants and breath fresheners are readily available. However, anyone suffering from serious and constant bad breath should seek medical advice.

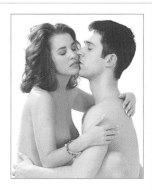

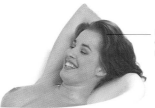

Lie back and enjoy being pampered

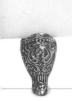

BATHING

Giving each other a bath, or sharing a shower, is not only cleansing and refreshing but also gets you in the mood for love. A tub or shower can also be an exciting place to make love.

11

EROGENOUS ZONES

Without imagination, sex can become boring and routine, and that is why it is often said that the brain is the most important of our sex organs. What all good lovers have, whether they be male or female, is a sensitive awareness of the erogenous zones—the areas of the body that generate sexual arousal when stimulated. By exploring these zones, you can make your lovemaking into a whole-body experience rather than one that is confined to the genitals.

THE EROGENOUS FOOT

According to the theory of reflexology, the feet are connected with the rest of the body by energy channels. When the feet are stimulated by touch, kissing, or massage, the enjoyable sensations that are created within them spread throughout the body.

Most women find gentle kissing and stroking of their breasts and nipples highly arousing

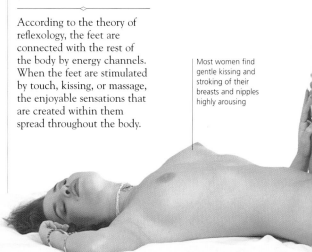

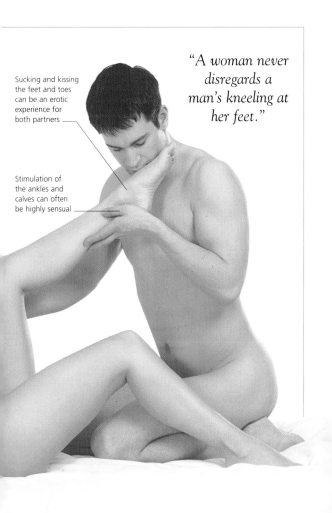

Sucking and kissing the feet and toes can be an erotic experience for both partners

Stimulation of the ankles and calves can often be highly sensual

"A woman never disregards a man's kneeling at her feet."

THE SENSUAL SKIN

The skin is the human body's largest single organ: an average adult has about 18 square feet (1.7 square meters) of skin, weighing around 6.6 lb (3 kilograms) and richly endowed with sensitive nerve endings. These nerve endings respond to the slightest touch and to the smallest changes in temperature or pressure. The skin on some parts of the body, however, is more sensitive to touch and other external stimuli than it is on others, the numerous erogenous zones being among those areas that are particularly sensitive.

THE BREASTS

Having their breasts gently squeezed and their nipples rubbed and kissed is more important to most women than many men realize.

The nipples are highly sensitive to touch, and some women can reach orgasm by manual or oral stimulation of the nipples alone.

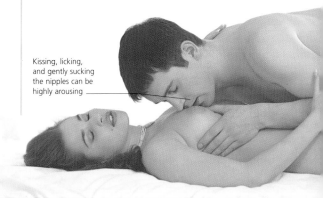

Kissing, licking, and gently sucking the nipples can be highly arousing

THE BUTTOCKS

For most men, a woman's buttocks act both as an attractor—because they enclose the genitals—and as a source of pleasure in themselves. It can be mutually stimulating if the man squeezes, rubs, and lightly slaps them, as well as kissing and biting them gently.

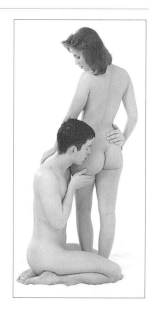

A man's buttocks, like those of a woman, can be highly responsive to sensual touch

CREATING THE MOOD

Careful preparation of the room in which you are going to make love is as important as preparing your body for lovemaking. Make sure that the room is at a comfortable temperature, provide background music that enhances the mood, and, to avoid unwanted interruptions, switch on your answering machine or unplug the phone.

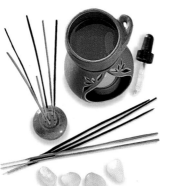

SCENTING THE ROOM
Use incense, heated essential oils, or scented crystals to give your bedroom an exotic, seductive scent.

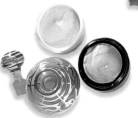

OILS AND LOTIONS
Smooth scented massage oils and lotions into each other's skin to make your foreplay more seductive.

THE SETTING FOR LOVE

Although the world has changed considerably since the days in which the Kama Sutra was written, when preparing for love it is still worth heeding the advice of Vatsyayana, who recommends that the room, "balmy with rich perfumes, should contain a bed, soft, agreeable to the sight, covered with a clean white cloth, having garlands and bunches of flowers upon it, and two pillows, one at the top, another at the bottom. There should also be a sort of couch besides, and at the head of this a sort of stool, on which should be placed the fragrant ointments for the night, as well as flowers, fragrant substances, and things used for perfuming the mouth."

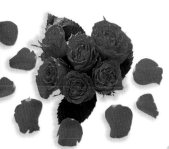

FLOWERS
Decorate and perfume your room with fresh, fragrant flowers, such as roses.

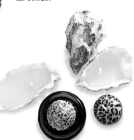

SOFT LIGHTING
The gentle, flickering glow of candlelight is much more romantic than electric light.

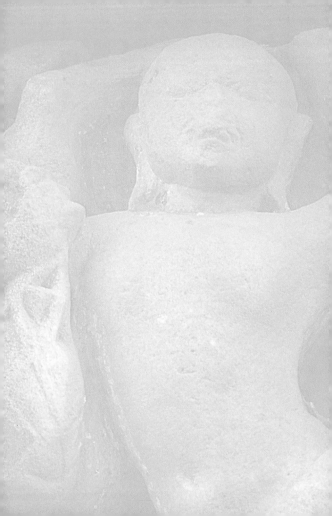

TOUCHING
AND
EMBRACING

"Women, being of a tender nature, want tender beginnings."

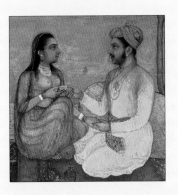

EMBRACING

The Kama Sutra describes the embraces depicted below and opposite as indicating "the mutual love of a man and woman." Those shown on pages 22–23 occur "at the time of the meeting," and those on pages 24–25 are "ways of embracing simple members of the body."

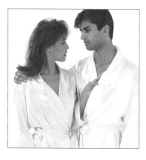

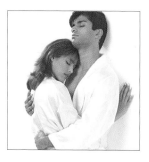

THE RUBBING
EMBRACE

THE PRESSING
EMBRACE

According to the *Kama Sutra*'s description, "When two lovers are walking slowly together, either in the dark, or in a place of public resort, or in a lonely place, and rub their bodies against each other, it is called a 'rubbing embrace.'"

The *Kama Sutra* sees this embrace as an extension of the Rubbing Embrace: "When on the above occasion [of the Rubbing Embrace] one of them presses the other's body forcibly against a wall or pillar, it is called a 'pressing embrace.'"

THE TOUCHING EMBRACE

In its description of this move, the *Kama Sutra* says that "When a man under some pretext or other goes in front or alongside of a woman and touches her body with his own, it is called the 'touching embrace.'" This embrace can, of course, be given by women as well as by men.

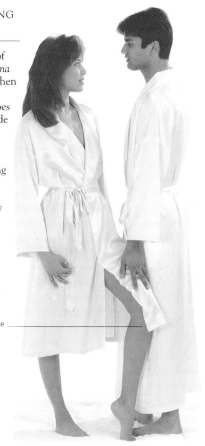

You can use your limbs and hands, as well as your body, for this embrace

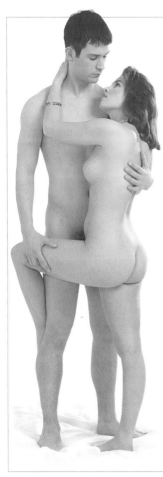

EMBRACING AND LOVEMAKING

Vatsyayana divides the embraces that are given at "the time of the meeting" into two groups. The first, which includes the Twining of a Creeper, consists of embraces used when the lovers are standing, but not in sexual union. The second group, including the other two embraces shown here, consists of those to be adopted during congress.

THE TWINING OF A CREEPER

The *Kama Sutra* describes this as "When a woman, clinging to a man as a creeper twines round a tree, bends his head down to hers with the desire of kissing him, embraces him, and looks lovingly toward him, it is called an embrace like the 'twining of a creeper.'"

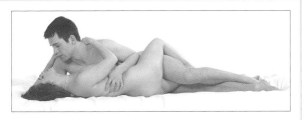

THE MIXTURE OF SESAMUM SEED WITH RICE

This embrace, described as being like "the mixture of sesamum [sesame] seed with rice," is what happens when lovers "embrace each other so closely that the arms and thighs of the one are encircled by the arms and thighs of the other."

THE MILK AND WATER EMBRACE

An embrace like a "mixture of milk and water" is what occurs when a man and woman "are very much in love with each other and, not thinking of any pain or hurt, embrace each other as if they were entering into each other's bodies either while the woman is sitting on the lap of the man, or in front of him, or on a bed."

THE AROUSAL OF MALE DESIRE

Quoting "some verses on the subject," the Kama Sutra says that "The whole subject of embracing is of such a nature that men who ask questions about it, or who hear about it, or who talk about it, acquire thereby a desire for enjoyment. Even those embraces that are not mentioned in the Kama Shastra [the Holy Writ of Kama] should be practiced at the time of sexual enjoyment, if they are in any way conducive to the increase of love or passion. The rules of the Shastra apply so long as the passion of man is middling, but when the wheel of love is once set in motion, there is then no Shastra and no order."

THE EMBRACE OF THE THIGHS

The Kama Sutra describes the "embrace of the thighs" as being "When one of two lovers presses forcibly one or both of the thighs of the other between his or her own."

Lovers move naturally on to intercourse from this position once both are fully aroused

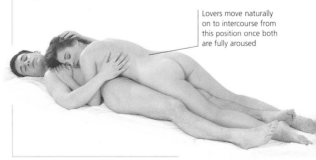

THE EMBRACE OF THE BREASTS

This is a form of upper-body contact that occurs when a man "places his breast between the breasts of a woman and presses her with it." This embrace stimulates the nipples of both partners simultaneously and is an arousing alternative to kissing the nipples or stimulating them manually.

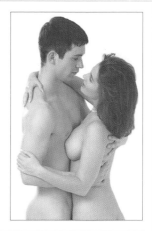

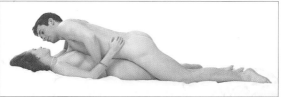

THE EMBRACE OF THE JAGHANA

The jaghana is the area between the navel and the thighs. When a man "presses the jaghana or middle part of the woman's body against his own, and mounts upon her to practice either scratching, or biting, or striking, or kissing, the hair of the woman being loose and flowing, it is called the 'embrace of the jaghana.'"

MUTUAL GROOMING

The Kama Sutra mentions the importance of bodily cleanliness, but not the great deal of shared pleasure that lovers can derive from mutual grooming, either for its own sake or in preparation for lovemaking. Mutual grooming can include taking a bath or shower together, shaving the man's face, and washing, drying, and brushing each other's hair. By delaying the act of love, it can heighten the anticipation of pleasure and encourage feelings of tenderness.

SHAVING

Vatsyayana recommends that a man shave his head and face every four days, and the other parts of his body every five to ten days. But no matter how sexy a woman may find her partner's stubble, she will probably not want to be scratched by it when they kiss. Instead of asking him to shave before making love, she could try shaving him herself.

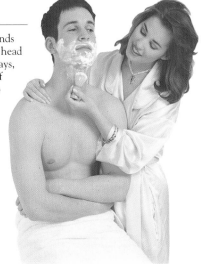

SHAMPOOING HER HAIR

As a prelude to lovemaking, shampooing is a sensuous form of mutual grooming. Many lovers enjoy washing and drying each other before going to bed, although this can simply be an affectionate part of a shared life, and need not always lead to sex.

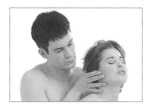

NECK MASSAGE
Help your lover relax by giving a gentle neck massage before shampooing her hair.

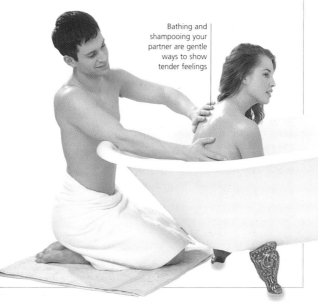

Bathing and shampooing your partner are gentle ways to show tender feelings

SENSUAL MASSAGE

The Kama Sutra, *surprisingly*, makes no mention of massage, although it has been widely used in the East for thousands of years. The aim of sensual massage, whether or not it is to end in lovemaking, is to relax both body and mind, so it is important to create a comfortable setting in which to give it. The room should be warm and softly lit, and you should try to ensure uninterrupted privacy.

BACK AND SPINE

Work upward from the buttocks, using gentle, erotic pressure. Keep your hands outspread and level with each other and your thumbs pushing always away from the spine. Work up to the base of the neck and out to the shoulders, and then down the sides to the buttocks.

Repeat this massage ten times or more, depending on your partner's wishes

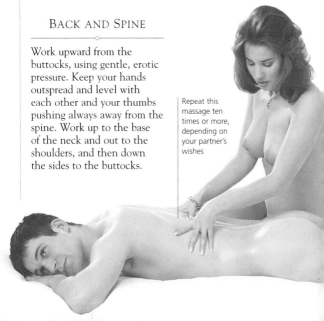

THE BASIC MASSAGE STROKES

The following basic massage strokes are effective and sensual, and, with a little practice, easy to perform.

Effleurage—*glide your palms across your partner's skin, putting your body weight behind the movement.*

Kneading—*gently curve your hands and knead the flesh with a smooth, regular movement.*

Pétrissage—*move the balls of your fingers or thumbs in circles alongside the spine to soothe away muscular tension.*

Hacking—*keeping your fingers relaxed, give a series of brisk chops with the side of the hand, as in karate but more softly.*

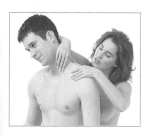

SHOULDERS AND HEAD

Begin by massaging the front of the shoulders, then work on the sides of the neck, the cheeks and the jaw, and the temples and forehead. Then run your fingers lightly over the chin, lips, eyes, and nose.

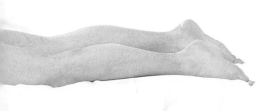

MASSAGE OILS AND ADDITIVES

You can give your partner a massage with dry hands, but your movements will be smoother and more effective, especially if you are inexperienced, if you use a massage oil or an oil-free massage lotion. There is a wide variety of suitable oils, many of them derived from nuts (particularly coconuts) or vegetables. Plain oils, such as almond, olive, grapeseed, and sunflower, can be used as base oils, perfumed by the addition of essential oils. Suitable essential oils to use include patchouli, sandalwood, ylang-ylang, jasmine, rose, lavender, rosemary, chamomile, cedarwood, and rosewood. To make up enough scented oil for one massage session, add up to a dozen drops of your chosen essential oil to about 1 fl oz (30 ml) of your base oil.

Using Massage Oil

The application of cold massage oil usually comes as a shock to the skin of the recipient. All massage oils work best when they have been prewarmed by rubbing them for a few seconds between the hands. Alternatively, you can warm the massage oil by standing the bottle in a bowl of hot water for a few minutes before you use it, and leaving it in the bowl between applications. Oil each area of your partner's skin just before you attend to it rather than oiling his or her whole body first: apply a small amount to the part you intend to massage, and rub it in with smooth but firm strokes. After the massage, you can either leave the oil to soak into your partner's skin, or you can remove it by wiping gently with a towel or by lovingly washing and drying the skin.

FEET AND LEGS

Start by massaging the toes and the areas between them. Next, run the palms of your hands firmly over the soles and tops of the feet, then move up the leg, working on the ankles, calves, and the backs of the thighs.

Massage her leg with one hand while holding it steady with the other

It is easier to massage your partner's feet, ankles, and calves if she lies face down

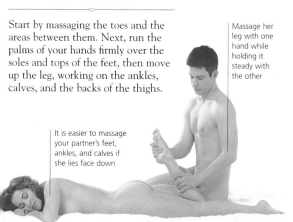

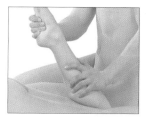

DOWNWARD LEG STROKES
Slide your hand down the leg from ankle to knee, squeezing the calf muscles firmly but gently with your fingertips.

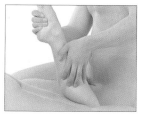

UPWARD LEG STROKES
Draw your hand back up from the knee to the ankle, using the same action as when making a downward stroke.

MASSAGE FOR SEXUAL AROUSAL

*To create arousal rather than relaxation when giving your
partner a sensual massage, switch from vigorous strokes to
very gentle actions. For example, if you trace a line back and
forth across your partner's breasts, nipples, and chest with
your fingertips, it can feel far more exciting for both of you
than the more forceful movements of conventional massage.*

*Many other areas of the body respond to an insistent,
"feathering" touch, including the neck, the insides of the arms
and thighs, the navel, the buttocks, and the calves. And you
need not restrict yourself to using your hands: try lying on
your partner and rubbing your body against his or hers.*

BUTTOCKS

Pressing firmly, move your
hands in a firm circular
motion over the buttocks.
Then press increasingly
lightly until your hands are
just brushing the skin. Finish
by kneading and squeezing
each buttock in turn.

Lean on your
hands when
you want to
apply firm
pressure

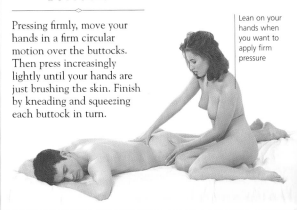

THE RITUALIZED BLOWS OF LOVE

The Kama Sutra describes a number of styles of harmless ritual striking that can be used by partners to heighten their excitement before and during intercourse. Four kinds of light blow are detailed: using the back of the hand; the fingers, slightly contracted; the fist; and the palm of the hand. These blows are said to be most effective when used on on the shoulders, the head, the space between the breasts, the back, the midriff, and on the sides. Modern lovers might use light blows on each other spontaneously, and aficionados of spanking will tell you that it can be very arousing.

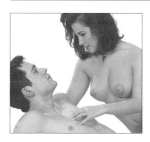

SCRATCHING

Using the fingernails to mark each other's skin during foreplay and lovemaking is not to everyone's taste, but the *Kama Sutra* regards them as a useful weapon in a lover's armory. And if scratching is based on passion rather than anger or cruelty, both partners may find that leaving love marks on each other's skin can be fun.

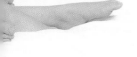

HAIR PLAY

The eternal fascination that a woman's hair has for a man, especially when it is long, is acknowledged by the Kama Sutra. It states that one of the arts a woman should learn is that of "dressing the hair with unguents and perfumes and braiding it." The erotic power of her hair is reciprocated when, by admiring and fondling it, her partner arouses feelings of desire in her, which he then undertakes to satisfy.

A LIGHT TOUCH

When a woman has long hair, it can fall beguilingly over her face or breasts and brush sensually against her partner's naked body. To arouse him further, she can kneel astride him and sweep it teasingly over his whole body, including his penis, so heightening his desire.

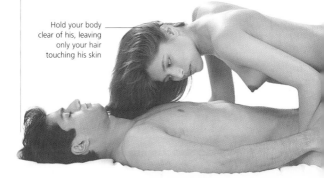

Hold your body clear of his, leaving only your hair touching your skin

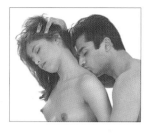

REVEALING THE NECK

A woman's clean, lustrous hair can be a powerful aphrodisiac, inviting her lover to toy with it and bury his face and hands in it. And when he lifts her hair to reveal a soft, delicate neck, his joy and arousal can be greatly intensified.

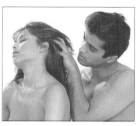

TACTILE PLEASURE

Both partners get pleasure when the man runs his fingers lovingly through the woman's hair. She can greatly increase the tactile pleasure for both of them—and enhance the eroticism of the situation—by doing the same thing to him.

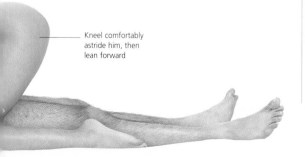

Kneel comfortably astride him, then lean forward

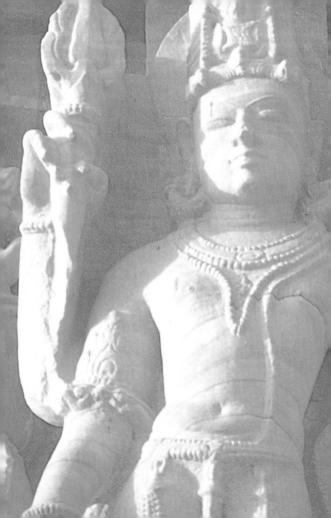

KISSING
AND
FOREPLAY

*"If the woman kisses
him, he should kiss
her in return."*

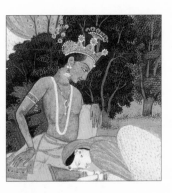

KISSING

The Kama Sutra recognizes kissing's power of expression by describing various types of kiss and suggesting when each type is appropriate. Kissing is an art in itself, and because the mouth is among the most sensitive parts of the body—and the most versatile—you can use your lips and tongue not only to kiss but also to lick, suck, nuzzle, or nibble any area of your partner's body.

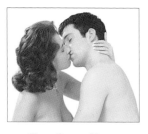

THE BENT KISS

This is the kind of kiss that occurs when "the heads of two lovers are bent toward each other, and when so bent, kissing takes place." It is one of the most natural and familiar ways to kiss your lover, and one that allows deep tongue penetration and maximum lip contact.

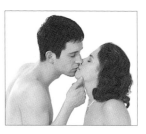

THE TURNED KISS

"When one of them turns up the face of the other by holding the head and chin, and then kissing, it is called a 'turned kiss,'" says the *Kama Sutra*. This kiss is ideal when you are making love slowly in a face-to-face standing or sitting position, or at the start of foreplay.

THE STRAIGHT KISS

The Straight Kiss is not usually an expression of intense passion, because tongue penetration is not practical when "the lips of two lovers are brought into direct contact with each other," with their heads angled very slightly to each side. This kiss is, however, a gentle way of showing affection and of displaying the initial stages of desire.

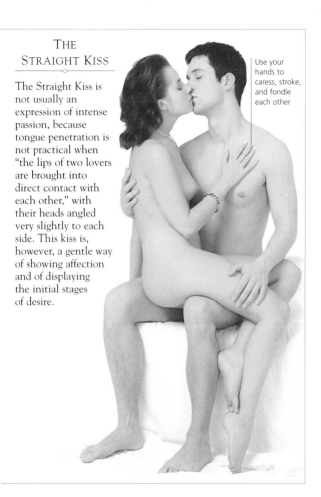

Use your hands to caress, stroke, and fondle each other

THE KISS OF THE UPPER LIP

The *Kama Sutra* says that when a man "kisses the upper lip of a woman, while she in return kisses his lower lip, it is called the 'kiss of the upper lip.'" This implies that the man initiates the kiss, but later on in its description of the arts of kissing, the book makes it clear that kisses can also be initiated by women.

Kiss your partner's upper and lower lips in turn to make this kiss more interesting

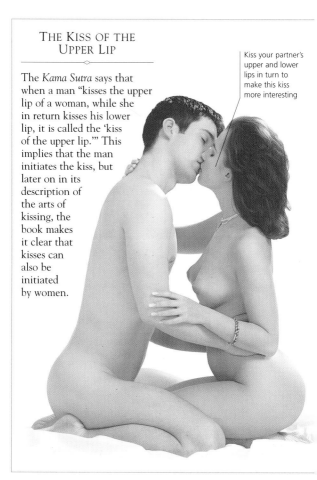

THE PRESSED KISS

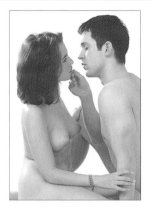

According to the *Kama Sutra*, in one version of this kiss "the lower lip is pressed with much force." A second variation, which is shown here, is "the greatly pressed kiss," in which one lover holds the other's lower lip, touches it with his or her tongue, and then kisses it with "great force."

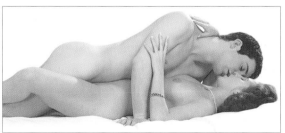

THE CLASPING KISS

The Clasping Kiss is what happens when either partner "takes both the lips of the other between his or her own." A woman, however, "only takes this kind of kiss from a man who has no mustache." This kiss can also involve the "fighting of the tongue," what we nowadays refer to as French kissing.

PLAYING THE KISSING GAME

The Kama Sutra describes a kissing game for lovers to play:

"As regards kissing, a wager may be laid as to which will get hold of the lips of the other first. If the woman loses, she should pretend to cry, should keep her lover off by shaking her hands, and turn away from him and dispute with him, saying, 'Let another wager be laid.' If she loses this a second time, she should appear doubly distressed, and when her lover is off his guard or asleep, she should get hold of his lower lip, and hold it in her teeth, and then she should laugh, make a loud noise, deride him, and say whatever she likes in a joking way. Such are the wagers as far as kissing is concerned."

Gently kiss your lover's back, neck, ears, cheeks, and lips

Use strokes and caresses to enhance your kissing

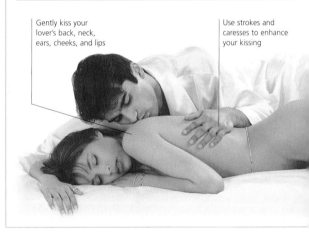

THE KISS
THAT TURNS AWAY

This is the kiss that a woman gives her lover when he is busy doing something else, so that "his mind may be turned away" from it. As most lovers are aware, a warm, lingering kiss (or kisses) can quickly take someone's mind off other things and direct it to thoughts of lovemaking.

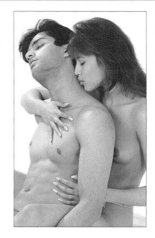

THE KISS THAT AWAKENS

According to the *Kama Sutra*, this is a kiss for a man to use on his partner late at night, when she is asleep, "to show her his desire. On such an occasion the woman may pretend to be asleep at the time of her lover's arrival, so that she may know his intention."

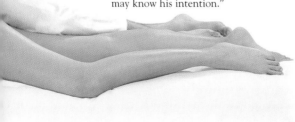

KISSING THE BODY

Most parts of the body, including the limbs, respond to kissing.
The lips and breasts are especially sensitive to the touch of
the mouth, but in general, the closer the kissing gets to the
genitals, the more intense and irresistible the pleasure—and
there is no need for either partner to remain passive. The
Kama Sutra, without giving details, says that the intensity of a
kiss should vary according to where on the body it is given,
and can be "moderate, contracted, pressed, or soft."

KISSING AND LICKING

Heighten anticipation of
lovemaking by covering your
partner's body with kisses,
licking it all over ("tongue
bathing"), and gently
nibbling it with your lips
and teeth. The greater your
self-control in delaying the
moment of penetration, the
greater will be the pleasure
for both of you when it
does occur.

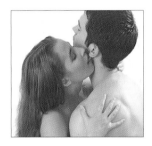

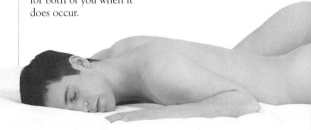

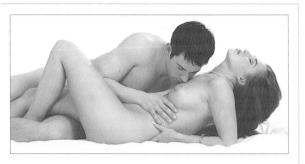

BREAST KISSING

When a man is kissing his partner's breasts, the most effective kisses will be those he applies lightly, and he should also gently kiss, suck, lick, or nibble her nipples. The nipples deserve special attention, because for many women, nipple stimulation is powerfully arousing.

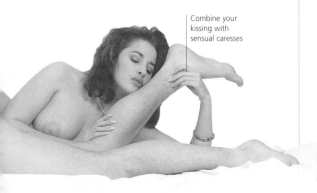

Combine your kissing with sensual caresses

◆ BITING

The Kama Sutra lists various types of bite in great detail and reflects an Indian erotic tradition in which biting is a vital part of the lover's repertoire. The bites it describes range from playful, teasing nips, through prolonged sucking that leaves a pronounced mark (a good definition of a love bite), to more intense biting at the height of passion. Most modern couples do not include the more forceful kinds of biting in their lovemaking, and they are sensible not to; at orgasm, the jaws may go into spasm and clamp shut, possibly inflicting a painful wound.

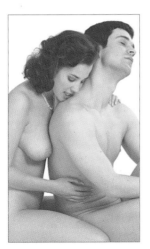

THE BITING OF A BOAR

The effect of this bite, intended for marking fleshy areas such as the breasts and shoulders, is described by the *Kama Sutra* as consisting of "many broad rows of marks near to one another, and with red intervals...This is impressed on the breasts and the shoulders; and these last two modes of biting are peculiar to persons of intense passion."

THE BITES OF LOVE

Eight different types of ritualized biting are listed in the Kama
Sutra. *In addition to the Biting of a Boar, these are:*

The Hidden Bite
*"The biting that is shown only by the excessive redness
of the skin that is bitten."*

The Swollen Bite
"When the skin is pressed down on both sides."

The Point
"When a portion of the skin is bitten with two teeth only."

The Line of Points
"When small portions of skin are bitten with all the teeth."

The Coral and the Jewel
*"The biting that is done by bringing together the teeth
and the lips is called the 'coral and the jewel.' The lip is
the coral, and the teeth the jewel."*

The Line of Jewels
*"When biting is done by all the teeth, it is called the
'line of jewels.'"*

The Broken Cloud
*"The biting that consists of unequal risings in a circle, and that
comes from the space between the teeth, is called the 'broken
cloud.' This is impressed on the breasts."*

CUNNILINGUS

The author of the Kama Sutra, Vatsyayana, reveals an ambivalent and rather coy attitude toward oral sex, concentrating on the pleasure the man gains from fellatio and discussing cunnilingus very briefly. This ambivalence possibly reflects the attitudes that were prevalent in his society. Even today, although oral sex is widely enjoyed and more freely discussed than in the past, many people of all ages (including those who are generally liberal and sexually active) disapprove of cunnilingus and fellatio, or at least never practice them. There are also many others who will consider fellatio but who disapprove of cunnilingus.

Lick and kiss her inner thighs as well as her perineum

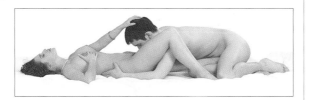

CLITORAL STIMULATION

Position yourself so that you can stroke your tongue upward over the shaft and head of her clitoris. Stimulate each side of the clitoris in turn, always from underneath, using featherlight strokes on its head and flicking the underside of its shaft from side to side with the tip of your tongue.

STIMULATING THE PERINEUM

Lie comfortably on your side with your head between her legs

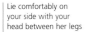

If your partner opens her legs wide, you can get your head between her thighs to lick her perineum, which is the area between her vagina and her anus. In most women, the perineum is rich in nerve endings and so it is very sensitive to being touched, stroked, or licked. This stimulation can be very exciting for a woman.

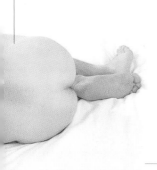

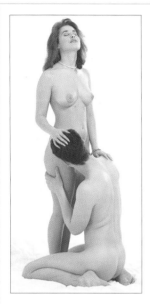

GENITAL KISSING

Try to create a slow—but highly erotic—crescendo of arousal when you give your lover oral sex. First kiss and lick her abdomen, her lower belly, and the insides of her thighs, and then slowly work in toward her genitals.

TONGUE INSERTION

To increase the stimulation after kissing and licking your lover's clitoris and perineum (*see page 51*), dart your tongue in and out of her vagina. Vary the strokes to give her an ever-changing range of sensations.

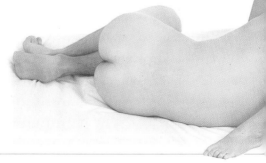

STIMULATION AND LUBRICATION

When a woman is sexually stimulated, her vagina produces a natural lubricating fluid. Cunnilingus is one of the best ways of stimulating her, and the resulting lubrication, in addition to allowing the vagina to receive a fully erect penis without discomfort, makes genital touch more pleasurable and full of sensuality for her. The stimulation does not have to be focused exclusively on the vagina itself, and the most erotic method of getting a woman to lubricate is through loving foreplay. Women who do not produce very much natural lubricant should use one of the water-soluble creams and jellies that are specially formulated as vaginal lubricants.

Relax and enjoy the erotic pleasure he is giving you

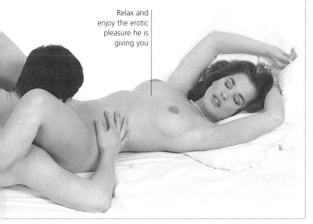

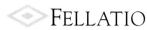

FELLATIO

The Kama Sutra describes fellatio—which it calls
Auparishtaka, or "mouth congress"—as an activity
predominantly practiced by eunuchs on their masters. It tells
how the duties of eunuchs, "disguised as females," included
pleasuring their masters with eight kinds of fellatio. These
days, gay men continue to enjoy the pleasures of fellatio,
and many heterosexual couples find it an arousing and
highly satisfying accompaniment to cunnilingus.

LICKING AND KISSING

When you start giving your
partner fellatio, hold the base
of his penis in one hand and
then, using the blade of your
tongue, repeatedly lick
upward. Lick slowly and
sensually first on one side of
his penis and then on the
other, as though it were an
ice-cream cone.

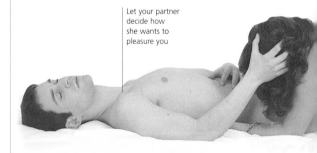

Let your partner
decide how
she wants to
pleasure you

THE BUTTERFLY FLICK

Flicking your tongue lightly along the ridge on the underside of your partner's penis is a highly effective fellatio technique. When you try this at first, you may need to hold the base of his penis. But with a little practice, you will be able to perform it without using your hands. This will leave them free to fondle and caress him.

Lie comfortably between your partner's legs

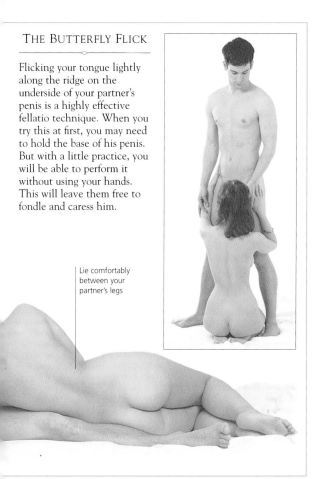

ORAL SEX ETIQUETTE

Always make sure that your penis is scrupulously clean before your partner gives you fellatio. And during it, be considerate and always let your partner know if you feel that you are about to climax. Then if she does not want you to ejaculate in her mouth she can withdraw your penis before you reach orgasm.

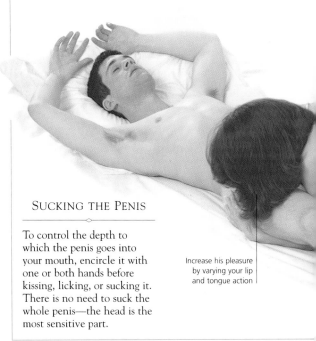

SUCKING THE PENIS

To control the depth to which the penis goes into your mouth, encircle it with one or both hands before kissing, licking, or sucking it. There is no need to suck the whole penis—the head is the most sensitive part.

Increase his pleasure by varying your lip and tongue action

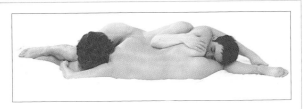

THE CONGRESS OF A CROW

The oral sex technique that the *Kama Sutra* calls the Congress of a Crow—"when a man and woman lie down in an inverted order, i.e., with the head of one toward the feet of the other and carry on this congress"—is the classic "Sixty-Nine" position, in which the two partners perform simultaneous fellatio and cunnilingus.

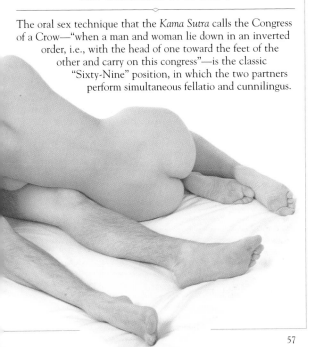

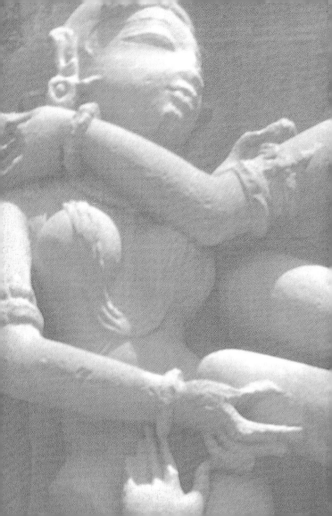

THE LOVE POSITIONS

"Congress having once commenced, passion alone gives birth to all the acts of the parties."

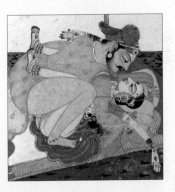

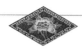

KAMA SUTRA
POSITIONS

Most people associate the *Kama Sutra* with exotic
descriptions of large numbers of impossible or even
bizarre lovemaking positions. In fact, very little of
the book is concerned directly with intercourse, and
it describes only about two dozen positions, most of
which are relatively easy to adopt if the woman is
reasonably supple. Vatsyayana, its author, lists eight
positions that had been described by an earlier
writer, Babhravya, and credits another early
author, Suvarnanabha, with the descriptions
of most of the rest. In most of the positions,
the woman lies on her back, but Vatsyayana
also suggests three woman-on-top styles of
lovemaking that can be used when a woman
"acts the part of a man."

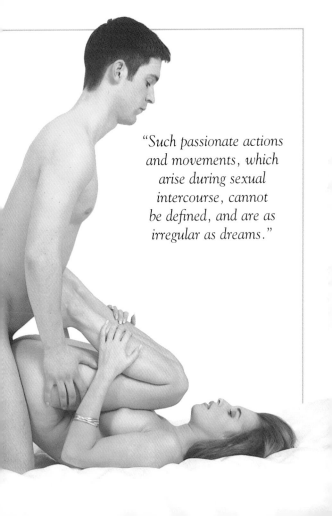

"Such passionate actions
and movements, which
arise during sexual
intercourse, cannot
be defined, and are as
irregular as dreams."

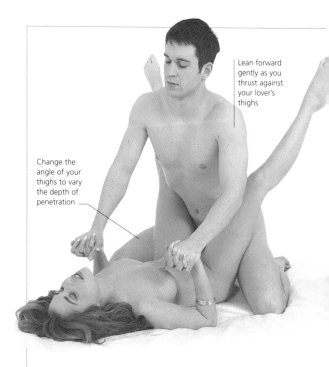

Lean forward gently as you thrust against your lover's thighs

Change the angle of your thighs to vary the depth of penetration

THE YAWNING POSITION

Lovers often adopt this posture spontaneously during lovemaking, especially when they have begun in a basic man-on-top position with their legs outstretched.

The woman raises and parts her thighs, and although the position does not allow for very deep penetration, this drawback is offset by its undeniable eroticism.

THE WIDELY OPENED POSITION

The woman arches her back and raises her body, opening her legs wide and supporting herself on her shoulders and feet. Because it gives her clitoris full exposure to the friction of intercourse, this position is likely to give the woman great stimulation.

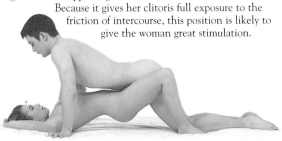

THE VARIANT YAWNING POSITION

Very deep and intensely pleasurable penetration is possible with this variation on the Yawning Position. Because of the extreme depth of penetration, the woman should be highly aroused before her partner enters her, and her vagina should be fully dilated.

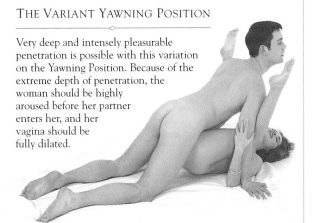

THE POSITION OF THE WIFE OF INDRA

The *Kama Sutra* says that this position is suitable for the "highest congress"—that is, lovemaking in which the vagina is fully open, thus ensuring maximum penetration. Achievable only by the loosest of limb, the position is named after Indrani, the beautiful and seductive wife of the Hindu deity Indra. In the early Vedic writings, he was the king of the gods and also the god of rain and thunder.

Bring your legs back as far as you can, then bend them at the knee

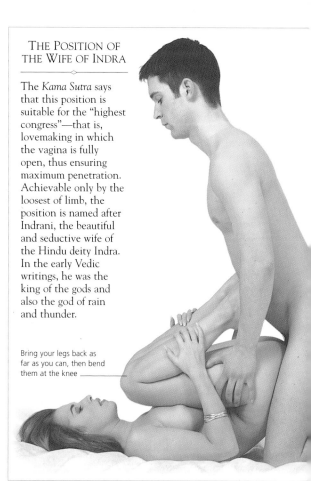

A MAN'S DUTY TO HIS PARTNER

The Kama Sutra places the obligation on the man to satisfy his partner, and offers suggestions on movements during love-making. These include: Moving Forward—ordinary penetration; Churning—holding and moving the penis in the vagina; Piercing—penetrating the vagina from above and pushing against the clitoris; Pressing—pushing the penis force-fully against the vagina; Blow of the Bull—rubbing one side of the vagina with the penis; Blow of the Boar—rubbing both sides of the vagina with the penis; Sporting of the Sparrow—moving the penis rapidly in and out of the vagina.

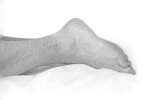

To help you control your thrusting, lean gently against your partner's feet and hold onto her thighs

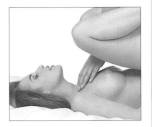

CARESSING HER BREASTS
In this position, you can reach down between your partner's knees to caress her breasts. When you do so, however, do not push hard against her feet because she will find that uncomfortable.

THE POWER OF TOUCH

Touch, along with other intimate forms of skin-to-skin contact, is an essential component of sexual activity and plays an important role in many other forms of human interaction. Good examples of nonsexual touch include handshakes and hugs. These are used as forms of greeting or farewell, and to express a variety of sentiments such as friendship, affection, love, sympathy, and congratulations. Although these are simple gestures, the precise way in which they are given tells the recipient a great deal about the intentions of the giver.

SIDE-BY-SIDE CLASPING POSITION

The *Kama Sutra* suggests that when adopting this gentle, relaxed, side-by-side version of the Clasping Position (*see opposite*), the man should always lie on his left side and the woman on her right. But whichever side they choose, most lovers enjoy the gentle intimacy of this posture.

Each partner's legs are outstretched and wrapped around the other's

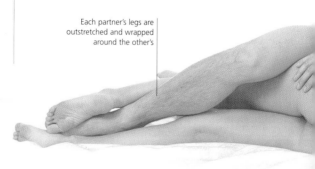

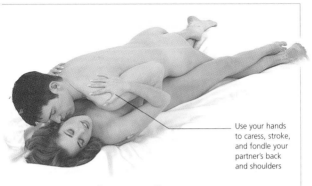

Use your hands to caress, stroke, and fondle your partner's back and shoulders

CLASPING POSITION

In the Clasping Position, the woman lies on her back and her partner lies over her with his legs entwined with hers. This position is really more of a loving, intimate embrace than a posture for active lovemaking, because the intertwined limbs tend to restrict movement.

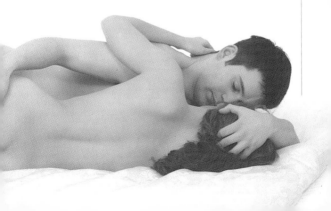

THE CHAKRAS: CENTERS OF ENERGY

In the yogic tradition (which had long been in existence by the time the Kama Sutra was written), the chakras are centers of energy that occur at seven points in the astral body, which the yogis believe surrounds and permeates the physical body. Six chakras are located along the astral equivalent of the spine, while the seventh crowns the head. Sexual activity is one way of arousing the energy known as kundalini, which lies dormant at the base of the spine and is often depicted as a coiled serpent. When aroused, it travels up through, and energizes, the chakras, revitalizing body and spirit.

THE PRESSING POSITION

During lovemaking, partners often slip effortlessly from one position to another, for instance from the Clasping Position *(see page 67)* to the Pressing Position. In this position, the woman grips her partner's thighs with hers so as to tighten her vagina around his penis.

Take your weight on your arms

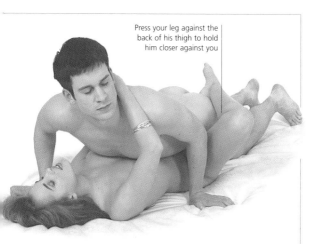

Press your leg against the
back of his thigh to hold
him closer against you

Use your hands to
caress your partner's
arms and body

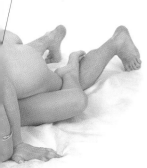

THE TWINING POSITION

A woman can use this
variation on the Pressing
Position (*see opposite*) to
express her desire for him by
wrapping herself closely about
him. In this position, she
places one leg across the back
of her lover's thigh and draws
him closer to her.

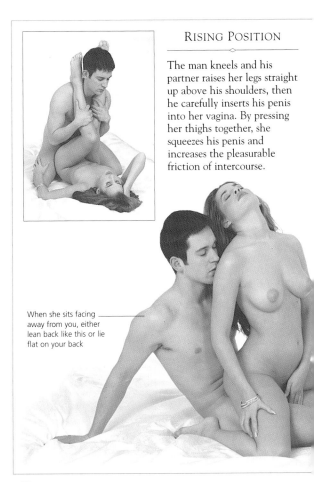

RISING POSITION

The man kneels and his partner raises her legs straight up above his shoulders, then he carefully inserts his penis into her vagina. By pressing her thighs together, she squeezes his penis and increases the pleasurable friction of intercourse.

When she sits facing away from you, either lean back like this or lie flat on your back

PRACTICING THE KEGEL EXERCISES

*These exercises are named after American gynecologist
Dr. A. H. Kegel. A woman can use them to tone her PC
(pubococcygeal) muscles and improve her vaginal response. To
locate your PC muscles, practice stopping the flow of urine
when you go to the bathroom: the muscles that you use to do
this are your PC muscles. The main Kegel exercise consists of
contracting the PC muscles for three seconds, relaxing them
for three seconds, and then repeating. Try doing this ten times,
on three separate occasions every day. When you become
proficient at this, do the exercise faster so that your vagina
"flutters." Do this ten times, three times a day.*

THE MARE'S POSITION

This is a very arousing and erotic technique that can be used in various lovemaking positions. The woman employs her vaginal muscles (those that contract at orgasm) to squeeze the penis as if milking it. This produces highly pleasurable sensations in both vagina and penis.

Sit in a relaxed position so
that you are not distracted
by discomfort in your legs

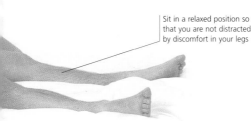

THE PRESSED
POSITION

The woman draws
her thighs back to
her chest, bends her
legs at the knee, and
places the soles of
both feet against
her partner's chest.
Her vagina is
shortened when
she is in this
position, so her
partner must be
careful with the
depth and force of
penetration to avoid
causing her pain as
he thrusts.

Push the soles of
your feet against
him, and press
your toes into
his chest

Hold on to her
legs to help you
control your
thrusting

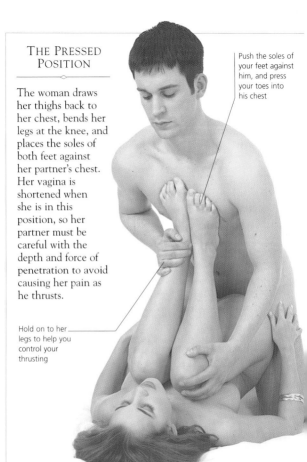

THE HALF-PRESSED POSITION

In this version of the Pressed Position (see *opposite*), the woman stretches one leg straight out and bends the other leg at the knee, placing the sole of her foot on his chest. As in the Pressed Position, the man should be careful not to thrust too hard.

If your leg gets tired, bend it at the knee and rest your heel on his buttocks

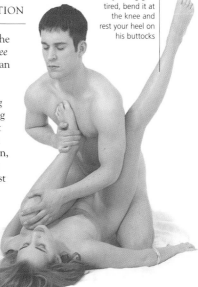

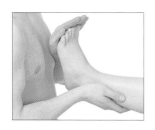

FOOT MASSAGE
Foot massage benefits the whole body (see page 12) and is also highly erotic. Massage both of your partner's feet, and then hold each foot behind the ankle with one hand and rotate it slowly with the other.

ACROBATIC POSITIONS

The lovemaking postures shown here and on the following two pages form a sequence of rather acrobatic positions. Because they are all somewhat difficult, I think that they should be approached in a spirit of fun rather than for excitement or eroticism.

THE SPLITTING OF A BAMBOO

Although this position is essentially a variant of the basic man-on-top posture, it requires considerably more suppleness from the woman. She raises one leg and puts it on her partner's shoulder for a time, then brings that leg down and raises the other. This sequence can be repeated over and over again.

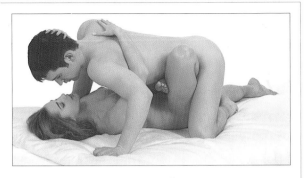

THE LOTUSLIKE POSITION

The woman draws in her legs and folds one over the other as neatly as possible, imitating the familiar yoga posture. In this position, her vagina is pulled up to meet her partner's penis.

Most women who try this difficult position find that they cannot hold it for long, if at all.

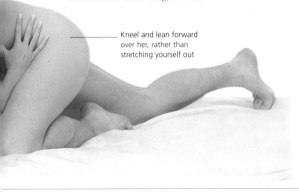

Kneel and lean forward over her, rather than stretching yourself out

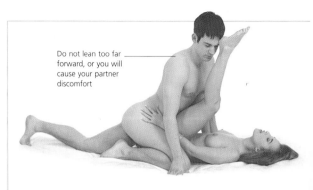

Do not lean too far forward, or you will cause your partner discomfort

FIXING OF A NAIL

This position is similar to the Splitting of a Bamboo (*see page 74*), but the woman places her heel against her partner's forehead instead of on his shoulder. Her leg and foot then symbolize a hammer driving in a nail, represented by his head.

Kneel comfortably between your partner's thighs

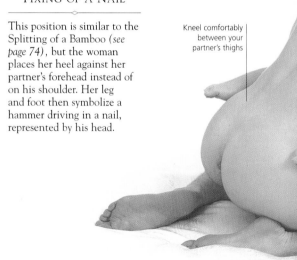

THE CRAB'S POSITION

In this position, the woman
bends and draws in both legs
and rests her thighs on her
stomach, rather like a crab
retracting its claws; this
tightens the vagina around
the penis. The man thrusts
from a kneeling position,
being careful not to penetrate
his partner too deeply.

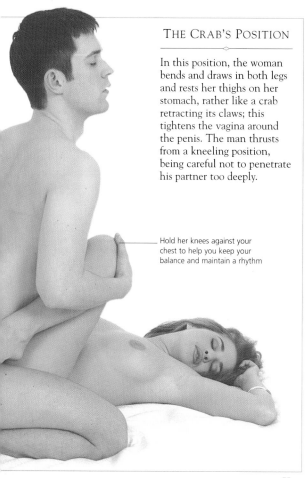

Hold her knees against your
chest to help you keep your
balance and maintain a rhythm

THE TURNING POSITION

This is a sequence of movements rather than a single position, and according to the *Kama Sutra* it can be learned "only by practice." It is an imaginative variant of the basic man-on-top position, and involves the man turning in a complete circle while maintaining penetration of his partner.

FIRST STAGE
Begin in the basic man-on-top ("missionary") position. The man lies with his legs between his partner's.

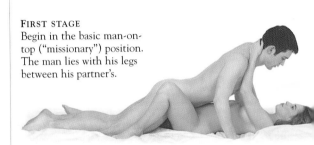

SECOND STAGE
Without withdrawing his penis, the man lifts first his left leg and then his right leg over his partner's right leg.

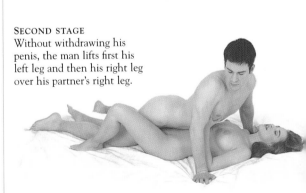

THIRD STAGE
Supporting himself on his arms, the man moves both legs around, again without withdrawing, until his body is at a right angle to hers.

It will be easier for him to keep his penis inside your vagina if your legs are slightly apart

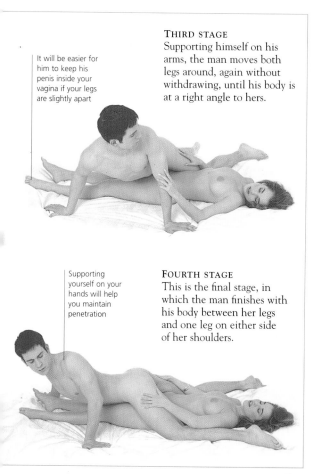

Supporting yourself on your hands will help you maintain penetration

FOURTH STAGE
This is the final stage, in which the man finishes with his body between her legs and one leg on either side of her shoulders.

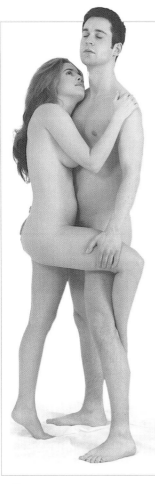

EROTIC SCULPTURES

The *Kama Sutra* and other classic Eastern love texts placed great emphasis on making love in standing positions. These positions are also more common than other postures in the erotic sculptures that traditionally adorned temple walls, an indication of the special status that they enjoyed.

THE SUPPORTED CONGRESS

The support referred to in this position's name is achieved by the lovers bracing themselves against each other, as shown here, or by one of them—usually the woman—leaning against a wall. Many couples find that leaning on a wall is better, because with the woman firmly supported by it, the man finds it easier to thrust vigorously.

THE SUSPENDED CONGRESS

To adopt this position, the man leans against a wall while his partner puts her arms around his neck. He then lifts her by holding her thighs or by locking his hands beneath her buttocks. If she is light, he may be able to support her with one arm around her waist, leaving the other hand free to stroke and caress her.

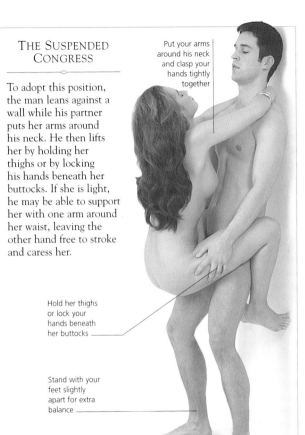

Put your arms around his neck and clasp your hands tightly together

Hold her thighs or lock your hands beneath her buttocks

Stand with your feet slightly apart for extra balance

WOMAN-ON-TOP POSITIONS

During lovemaking, the woman may often adopt a position on top of her partner. She might do this as a matter of personal preference, or when her partner is beginning to tire but she is still not satisfied. The *Kama Sutra* recommends three movements for her to use: the Top, shown here, the Swing, and the Pair of Tongs (*see pages 84–85*).

FIRST STAGE
Start in the basic woman-on-top position, then turn to face his feet.

Use your hands to help you keep your balance

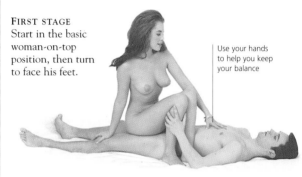

THE TOP

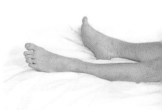

While sitting astride her partner, the woman raises her legs to clear his body and then swivels carefully around on his penis so that she faces first his feet and then eventually his head again. According to Vatsyayana, this movement requires considerable practice.

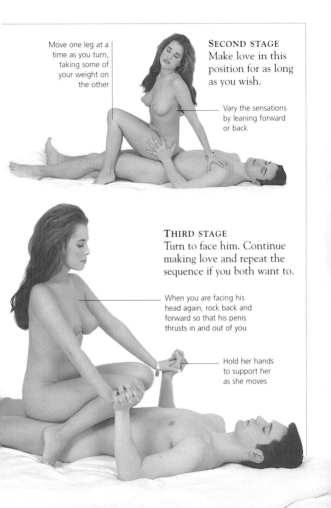

Move one leg at a
time as you turn,
taking some of
your weight on
the other

SECOND STAGE
Make love in this
position for as long
as you wish.

Vary the sensations
by leaning forward
or back

THIRD STAGE
Turn to face him. Continue
making love and repeat the
sequence if you both want to.

When you are facing his
head again, rock back and
forward so that his penis
thrusts in and out of you

Hold her hands
to support her
as she moves

THE PAIR OF TONGS

The man lies flat on his back, and the woman sits astride and facing him with her legs bent at the knee. She then draws his penis into her and holds it tight for a long time, repeatedly squeezing it with the muscles of her vagina; penetration is deep. This posture is perhaps the most practical of the three woman-on-top positions suggested by the *Kama Sutra*.

Lean forward or back to vary the angle of penetration

Lie back and enjoy the pleasure she is giving you, or thrust upward to increase your mutual excitement

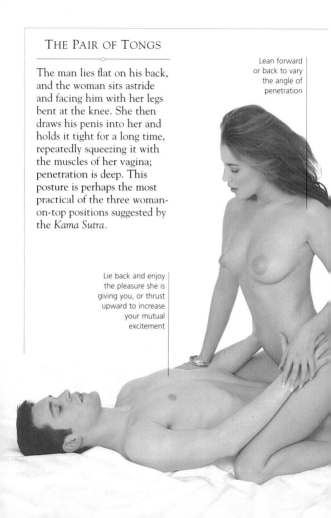

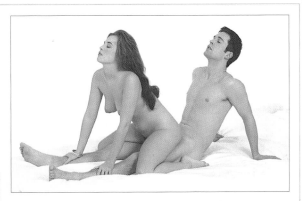

THE SWING

For this variation on the Top (*see page 82*), the *Kama Sutra* suggests that the man should lie with his back arched while the woman moves on top of him, but this is only feasible if the man is strong enough. It is usually easier for him to lie flat on his back while she is actually turning.

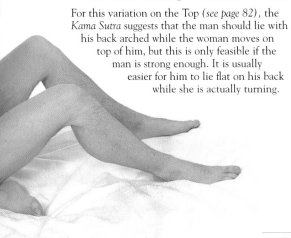

THE POWER OF IMAGINATION

The impossibility of listing every possible lovemaking position is acknowledged by Vatsyayana, who suggests instead that imaginative lovers can extend their repertoires by seeking inspiration from the animal kingdom. After his description of the Congress of a Cow, Vatsyayana says that "In the same way can be carried on the congress of a dog, the congress of a goat, the congress of a deer, the forcible mounting of an ass, the congress of a cat, the jump of a tiger, and the mounting of a horse. And in all these cases the characteristics of these different animals should be manifested by acting like them."

THE ELEPHANT POSTURE

The woman lies face down on the bed, and her partner lies over her with the small of his back arched inward. Once he is inside her, she can intensify the sensations for both of them by pressing her thighs closely together.

CONGRESS OF A COW

This is a variation on the more common rear-entry postures in which the woman kneels. Here, she supports herself on her hands and feet and her partner "mounts her like a bull." Deep penetration is possible in this position.

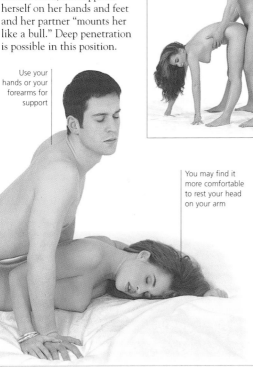

Use your hands or your forearms for support

You may find it more comfortable to rest your head on your arm

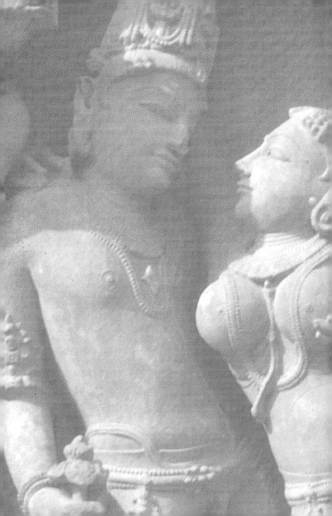

SAFER SEX
AND LOVING
AFTERPLAY

*"Those things which
increase passion
should be done first."*

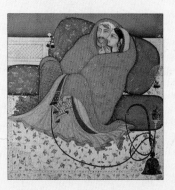

SAFER SEX

Although people have always tried to avoid catching sexually transmitted diseases, such as gonorrhea and syphilis, the practice of "safer sex" is very recent. This change in sexual behavior has been brought about by the spread of AIDS (Acquired Immune Deficiency Syndrome). The term "safer sex" describes sexual activity that is unlikely to lead to infection by HIV (the Human Immunodeficiency Virus), which is the cause of AIDS. The most common way in which the virus is passed is through the exchange of bodily fluids (semen, vaginal secretions, and blood).

NONPENETRATIVE SEX

Penetration need not occur every time a couple have sex. Embracing, stroking, and massage all express closeness, with only minimal risk of HIV infection. Masturbation may be used in the same way, if care is taken to avoid contact with bodily fluids.

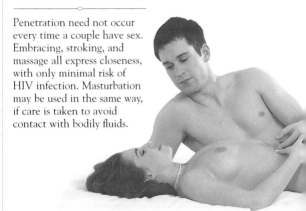

HIV AND THE DEVELOPMENT OF AIDS

*When it gets into the bloodstream, HIV progressively destroys
the immune system, the complex mechanism that enables the
body to defend itself against disease. This eventually leaves the
body vulnerable to other infections, including otherwise rare
illnesses such as certain types of cancers and pneumonias. A
person with HIV is said to have developed AIDS when he or
she begins to be affected by such illnesses, and it is these, not
the HIV infection itself, that will eventually cause the
death of a person with AIDS.*

Minimizing risk

*To reduce the risk of contracting HIV during intercourse
with a partner who may be infected, use a latex condom
(see page 92) in combination with a spermicide, preferably
one that contains nonoxynol-9. Always use condoms
during fellatio and latex "dental dams" during cunnilingus
to prevent contact with bodily fluids.*

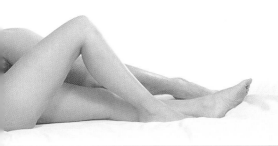

CONDOMS

The condom plays a crucial role in the practice of safer sex, because it substantially reduces the risk of HIV infection and offers effective protection against other sexually transmitted diseases (and against pregnancy). If you turn the task of putting on the condom into an erotic experience for both of you, it will not interrupt the flow of your lovemaking. And any loss of sensation resulting from use of a condom is a small price to pay for protection against HIV and other infections.

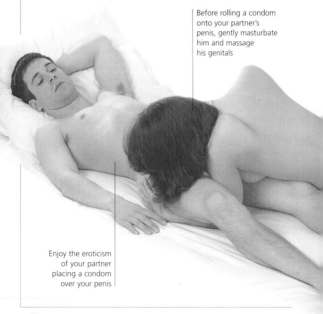

Before rolling a condom onto your partner's penis, gently masturbate him and massage his genitals

Enjoy the eroticism of your partner placing a condom over your penis

CHOOSING AND USING YOUR CONDOMS

To be effective, condoms must be of dependable quality, so avoid obscure brands and check the use-by date. Never reuse a condom, and be careful to avoid bringing one into contact with any oil-based product such as massage oil or cream, baby oil, or petroleum jelly. This is because condoms are made of latex, a material that is easily damaged and weakened by even the briefest contact with oil or an oil-based product. If you need to use a lubricant during intercourse, use a water-based product such as K-Y Jelly. Some people dislike using condoms, but this is a learned aversion that is relatively easy to unlearn. As an alternative, you could try using female condoms, which fit into the vagina rather than over the penis.

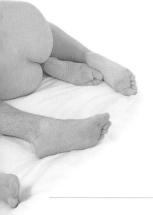

USING A CONDOM

After removing the condom from its foil packet, squeeze the air from the tip by holding it between your forefinger and thumb (air trapped inside could cause it to split during use). Then use slow, sensuous movements to roll it into place. If your partner is uncircumcised, ease back his foreskin before unrolling the condom.

Prolong the Mood

After making love, partners who genuinely care for each other will want to stay close emotionally and physically so as to prolong the unique closeness that lovemaking brings. Some lovers find that, having just reaffirmed a continuing intimate bond by making love, they can talk more easily about things that matter to them either as a couple or as individuals. They take this opportunity to discuss what they enjoy most about their sexual relationship, and feel free to tell each other if there is anything about their lovemaking that they would like to change. Often, though, a couple will want to make love again, in which case the woman might need to masturbate her partner to get him erect again. If they do not intend to resume lovemaking, but the woman was not able to reach a satisfactory climax, the considerate thing for her lover to do would be to help her achieve orgasm by masturbating her.

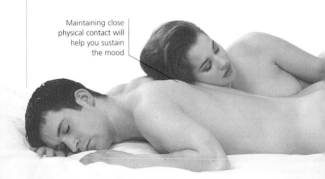

Maintaining close physical contact will help you sustain the mood

WHAT TO DO AFTERWARD

The Kama Sutra advises on the sensual delights that partners should share after making love: "At the end of the congress, the lovers with modesty, and not looking at each other, should go separately to the washing room. After this, sitting in their own places, they should eat some betel leaves, and the citizen should apply with his own hand to the body of the woman some pure sandalwood ointment, or ointment of some other kind. He should then embrace her with his left arm, and with agreeable words should cause her to drink from a cup held in his own hand, or he may give her water to drink. They can eat sweetmeats, or anything else according to their likings."

SUSTAINING THE HARMONY

The warm glow that follows lovemaking is all too easily dissipated if you simply go to sleep, or do anything that is either physically or intellectually demanding. Most lovers want to sustain the feeling of harmony; some like simply to lie quietly in each other's arms, while others choose to get up but prolong the mood by enjoying an undemanding activity such as eating together.

INDEX